Contents

What is Gout?

Gout is a common type of arthritis that causes intense pain, swelling, and stiffness in a joint. It usually affects the joint in the big toe.

Gout attacks can come on quickly and keep returning over time, slowly harming tissues in the region of the inflammation, and can be extremely painful. Hypertension, cardiovascular, and obesity are risk factors for gout.

It is the most common form of inflammatory arthritis in men, and although it is more likely to affect men, women become more susceptible to it after the menopause.

The Centers for Disease Control and Prevention (CDC) report that 8.3 million Americans were affected by gout between 2007 to 2008.

Treatment

The majority of gout cases are treated with medication. Medication can be used to treat the symptoms of gout attacks, prevent future flares, and reduce the risk of gout complications such as kidney stones and the development of tophi.

Commonly used medications include nonsteroidal anti-inflammatory drugs (NSAIDs), colchicine, or corticosteroids. These reduce inflammation and pain in the areas affected by gout and are usually taken orally.

Medications can also be used to either reduce the production of uric acid (xanthine oxidase inhibitors such as allopurinol) or improve the kidney's ability to remove uric acid from the body (probenecid).

Without treatment, an acute gout attack will be at its worst between 12 and 24 hours after it began. A person can expect to recover within 1 to 2 weeks without treatment, but there may be significant pain during this period.

Tests and diagnosis

Gout can be tricky to diagnose, as its symptoms, when they do appear, are similar to those of other conditions. While hyperuricemia occurs in the majority of people that develop gout, it may not be present during a flare. On top of that, the majority of people with hyperuricemia do not develop gout.

One diagnostic test that doctors can carry out is the joint fluid test, where fluid is extracted from the affected joint with a needle. The fluid is then examined to see if any urate crystals are present.

As joint infections can also cause similar symptoms to gout, a doctor can look for bacteria when carrying out a joint fluid test in order to rule a bacterial cause. The fluid may need to be sent to a lab, where it can take several days to analyze.

Doctors can also do a blood test to measure the levels of uric acid in the blood, but, as mentioned, people with high uric acid levels do not always experience gout. Equally, some people can develop the symptoms of gout without having increased levels of uric acid in the blood.

Finally, doctors can search for urate crystals around joints or within a tophus using ultrasound scan. X-rays cannot detect gout, but may be used to rule out other causes.

Types

There are various stages through which gout progresses, and these are sometimes referred to as different types of gout.

Asymptomatic hyperuricemia

It is possible for a person to have elevated uric acid levels without any outward symptoms. At this stage, treatment is not required, though urate crystals may deposit in tissue and cause slight damage.

People with asymptomatic hyperuricemia may be advised to take steps to address any possible factors contributing to uric acid build-up.

Acute gout

This stage occurs when the urate crystals that have been deposited suddenly cause acute inflammation and intense pain. This sudden attack is referred to as a "flare" and will normally subside within 3 to 10 days. Flares can sometimes be triggered by stressful events, alcohol and drugs, as well as cold weather.

Interval or intercritical gout

This stage is the period in between attacks of acute gout. Subsequent flares may not occur for months or years, though if not treated, over time, they can last longer and occur more frequently. During this interval, further urate crystals are being deposited in tissue.

Chronic tophaceous gout

Chronic tophaceous gout is the most debilitating type of gout. Permanent damage may have occurred in the joints and the kidneys. The patient can suffer from chronic arthritis and develop tophi, big lumps of urate crystals, in cooler areas of the body such as the joints of the fingers.

It takes a long time without treatment to reach the stage of chronic tophaceous gout – around 10 years. It is very unlikely that a patient receiving proper treatment would progress to this stage.

Pseudogout

One condition that is easily confused with gout is pseudogout. The symptoms of pseudogout are very similar to those of gout, although thr flare-ups are usually less severe.

The major difference between gout and pseudogout is that the joints are irritated by calcium pyrophosphate crystals rather than urate crystals. Pseudogout requires different treatment to gout.

Causes

Gout is caused initially by an excess of uric acid in the blood, or hyperuricemia. Uric acid is produced in the body during the breakdown of purines – chemical compounds that are found in high amounts in certain foods such as meat, poultry, and seafood.

Normally, uric acid is dissolved in the blood and is excreted from the body in urine via the kidneys. If too much uric acid is produced, or not enough is excreted, it can build up and form needle-like crystals that trigger inflammation and pain in the joints and surrounding tissue.

Risk factors

There are a number of factors that can increase the likelihood of hyperuricemia, and therefore gout:

Age and gender: Men produce more uric acid than women, though women's levels of uric acid approach those of men after the menopause.

Genetics: A family history of gout increases the likelihood of the condition developing.

Lifestyle choices: Alcohol consumption interferes with the removal of uric acid from the body. Eating a high-purine diet also increases the amount of uric acid in the body.

Lead exposure: Chronic lead exposure has been linked to some cases of gout.

Medications: Certain medications can increase the levels of uric acid in the body; these include some diuretics and drugs containing salicylate.

Weight: Being overweight increases the risk of gout as there is more turnover of body tissue, which means more production of uric acid as a metabolic waste product. Higher levels of body fat also increase levels of systemic inflammation as fat cells produce pro-inflammatory cytokines.

Recent trauma or surgery: Increases risk.

Other health problems: Renal insufficiency and other kidney problems can reduce the body's ability to efficiently remove waste products, leading to elevated uric acid levels. Other conditions associated with gout include high blood pressure and diabetes.

Symptoms

Gout usually becomes symptomatic suddenly without warning, often in the middle of the night.

The main symptoms are intense joint pain that subsides to discomfort, inflammation, and redness.

Gout frequently affects the large joint of the big toe, but can also affect the forefoot, ankles, knees, elbows, wrists, and fingers.

The pain can be excruciating. A veteran visiting a Hospital in Birmingham, AL, said:

"I've been shot, beat up, stabbed, and thrown out of a helicopter, but none of that compared to the gout."

Complications

In some cases, gout can develop into more serious conditions, such as:

- Kidney stones: If urate crystals collect in the urinary tract, they can become kidney stones.

- Recurrent gout: Some people only ever have one flare up; others may have regular recurrences, causing gradual damage to the joints and surrounding tissue.

Prevention tips

There are many lifestyle and dietary guidelines that can be tried to protect against flares or prevent gout from occurring in the first instance:

- maintain a high fluid intake of around 2 to 4 liters a day

- avoid alcohol

- maintain a healthy body weight

Home remedies

Individuals with gout can manage flare-ups by moderating their diet. A balanced diet can help reduce symptoms.

Decreasing foods that are high in purines, to ensure that the levels of uric acid in the blood do not get too high, is reasonable to try. Here is a list of high-purine foods to be wary of:

- anchovies

- asparagus

- beef kidneys

- brains

- dried beans and peas

- game meats

- gravy

- herring

- liver

- mackerel

- mushrooms

- sardines

- scallops

- sweetbreads

While it is reasonable to decrease or avoid these foods, it has been found that a high purine-rich diet does not increase the risk of gout, or aggrevate symptoms in research studies.

Asparagus, beans, some other plant-based foods, and mushrooms are also sources of purines, but research suggests that these do not trigger gout attacks and do not impact uric acid levels.

Various epidemiological studies have shown that purine-rich vegetables, whole grains, nuts and legumes, and less sugary fruits, coffee, and vitamin C supplements lower blood uric acid levels, but do not decrease the risk of gout. Red meat, fructose-containing beverages, and alcohol can increase the risk.

The role of uric acid in gout has been clearly defined and understood. As a result of this and the wide availability of relevant medications, gout is a very controllable form of arthritis.

Gout Diet

A well-balanced gout diet can not only lower your risk of an attack, but it can also slow the progression of gout-related joint damage. The key is to choose foods that are low in purine a chemical compound that, when metabolized, creates the uric acid that triggers gout attacks. Purine is found in many foods, like organ meats, beer, and soda, so these are avoided. Nutritious foods that help your body eliminate uric acid are at the center of an effective diet for managing gout.

A gout diet is generally part of a comprehensive program recommended after you have been diagnosed with the condition. You'll work together with your healthcare provider to manage several lifestyle factors, including diet, weight control, physical activity, and possibly medication to reduce the frequency and intensity of gout attacks.

Benefits

In the human body, purines are either endogenous (made by the body) or exogenous (consumed in food). When exogenous purines are broken down by the liver, a waste product called uric acid is created. It is normally excreted, but that is not the case when you have gout. The condition, in fact, is defined by the build-up of uric acid.

For centuries, gout has been associated with the overindulgence of rich foods such as seafood, meat, and alcohol. As a result, people were commonly advised to avoid all of these things until symptoms resolved.

With the discovery of purines in 1884, the practice was further endorsed, and people were routinely warned against consuming otherwise healthy foods such as fish, vegetables, and fruit because they contained the chemical as well.

In recent years, however, understanding of the synthesis of uric acid has expanded considerably, and many of the plant-based high-purine foods once considered off-limits are today deemed safe for consumption.

This knowledge has allowed the gout diet to evolve to be more nutritious while still being helpful in managing this condition.

According to the American Academy of Rheumatology, gout treatment may include medication and lifestyle changes. The organization emphasizes that treatment should be tailored for each individual. What works for one person may be less effective for another.

But studies have shown that following a gout diet can improve the frequency of gout attacks and reduce the severity of symptoms in some people. In fact, a study published in Annals of the Rheumatic Diseases found that consuming a purine-rich diet increased the risk of recurrent gout attacks fivefold among gout patients, whereas avoiding or reducing purine-rich foods (especially of animal origin) helped reduce the risk of gout attacks.

Following a lower purine diet may also help some people achieve and maintain a healthy weight. This is important in relation to gout because it not only can reduce the risk of developing the condition, but it can reduce pressure on the joints, help reduce pain, improve function, and slow the progression of arthritis issues that those diagnosed with gout are often faced with.

How It Works

On a gout diet, you'll try to avoid most foods that are rich in purines, especially from animal and seafood sources. Purine-rich vegetables do not increase your risk of a gout attack and can be consumed. Moderate portions of foods that are rich in vitamin C, low-fat dairy products, and plant oils should also be consumed to help manage your condition.

Duration

There is no cure for gout. As such, adopting the gout diet can be a part of your long-term care plan to help you spend more time in remission and less time managing painful flare-ups.

What to Eat

Compliant Foods

- Vegetables

- Low-fat dairy

- Tofu

- Whole grains

- Beans and lentils

- Plant-based oils

- Citrus fruits

- Cherries

- Coffee

Non-Compliant Foods

- Red meat

- Organ meats

- Coldwater fish

- Some shellfish

- Yeast extract

- Beer, liquor

- Sugary foods and beverages

Vegetables: Recent evidence shows that consumption of purine-rich vegetables like asparagus, spinach, and cauliflower does not affect uric acid levels or increase the risk of a gout attack, as was once thought. Plus, eating a diet that includes plenty of vegetables helps you to reach and maintain a healthy weight and provides your body with important vitamins and minerals.

Low-fat dairy: Studies have shown that the proteins in dairy products can help reduce uric acid levels. Choosing low-fat products such as skim milk or low-fat yogurt will help you to maintain a healthy weight as well.

Tofu, whole grains, beans, and lentils: Plant-based proteins will help you maintain a balanced diet while managing your condition. On the gout diet, you reduce your intake of meat and seafood, but you'll still want to consume about 15% to 30% of your calories from protein to meet U.S. Department of Agriculture (USDA) recommendations. There is some evidence that plant-based proteins and plant-based oils (such as olive, sunflower, and soy) may even protect you against gout attacks.

Citrus fruit: Evidence has shown that a daily intake of 500 milligrams (mg) of vitamin C may be an effective way to reduce the frequency of gout flare-ups. Vitamin C helps your body to excrete uric acid, and citrus fruits are a great source of this essential nutrient. Try to choose lower-fructose fruits such as grapefruit, oranges, or pineapple, as this natural sugar can increase uric acid levels.

Cherries: Researchers have found that that cherry consumption lowers serum uric acid levels and can reduce the risk of flare-ups in gout patients. Cherries and some cherry products (such as tart cherry juice) also contain high levels of anthocyanins flavonoids with anti-inflammatory and antioxidant properties that are helpful in managing the pain and inflammation associated with gout attacks.

Red meat and organ meat: Red meats are higher in purines than white meat. Higher consumption of red meat (including beef, venison, bison) and organ meats (including liver, sweetbreads, tongue, and kidney) increases the risk of recurrent gout attacks.

Coldwater fish, shellfish: Certain types of fish are known to be higher in purines and should be limited on a gout diet. Coldwater fish such as tuna, sardines, and anchovies are higher in purine, as are shellfish including shrimp, oysters, crab, and lobster.

Yeast extract: Certain spreads including Marmite, Vegemite, and Vitam-R contain yeast extract and are known to be high in purine. Avoid these to reduce uric acid levels.

Sugary foods and beverages: Foods and beverages that contain fructose—particularly those that contain high fructose corn syrup—are not advised on a gout diet. Keep uric acid levels lower by limiting or avoiding consumption of sodas and other sugary drinks, canned fruit or fruit juice, and other products including snack bars, candy, and breakfast cereals.

Recommended Timing

There is no specific food schedule that you need to follow on a gout diet. You can time your meals and snacks as you normally would to provide steady energy throughout the day. However, if you take medications to manage pain (including over-the-counter or prescription medications), your healthcare provider may suggest that you take the medication with a snack or meal to ease stomach upset.

Also, give yourself time to adjust to the gout diet when you first begin. Working out which foods are safe for you can be a process of trial and error. For example, while some people will have no problem consuming moderate amounts of red meat, others may experience an attack with only a scant helping.

Cooking Tips

There are plenty of foods to enjoy on the gout diet. Organizing your kitchen and following a few basic cooking tips will help you stick to your plan.

- Cook grains and dried beans in advance: Whole grains usually take longer to cook than refined grains. And if you buy dried beans (which are often cheaper than canned ones), those take extra time to soak and cook as well. Take one day during the week to cook a big batch, then keep your beans refrigerated in single-serving containers to grab when you need them.

• Learn to use plant-based oils: Using oils like olive oil or sunflower oil are associated with a lower risk of gout and better management of uric acid levels. But some of these oils usually have a lower flash point, meaning that they start to smoke at a lower temperature. When using a plant-based oil for the first time, reduce the heat until you are comfortable cooking with it.

• Experiment with tofu: Soy-based protein sources, like tofu, are unfamiliar to many consumers. But this versatile food is easy to find in the refrigerated section of the grocery store and easy to use. Consider a tofu scramble for breakfast, or enjoy a crunchy lettuce wrap with tofu, vegetables, and brown rice for a savory lunch or dinner.

Modifications

Almost anyone can follow the gout diet. Vegetarians, vegans, and those who follow a gluten-free diet can adjust the eating plan according to their program. For example, those on a gluten-free diet would choose gluten-free grains such as quinoa. Those who follow a plant-based diet will have an easy time adjusting to the gout diet as it emphasizes vegetables and some fruits.

Those who follow a pescatarian diet or a Mediterranean diet may have a harder time on the gout diet because fish is limited on the plan. However, some experts, including those at the

Arthritis Foundation, suggest that consuming certain types of fish (such as salmon) occasionally may be beneficial.

Considerations

The gout diet is one that will need to become a way of life. Give yourself time to adjust to your new eating plan. As you do, keep these things in mind.

General Nutrition

When following the gout diet, you'll find it easy to meet nutritional recommendations established by the USDA. You are encouraged to fill your plate with healthy vegetables, fruit, lean meat (such as poultry), whole grains, and low-fat dairy, which are standard recommendations for everyone, regardless of whether or not they have your condition.

If you currently consume red meat as your primary source of protein, it may take some time to learn how to replace it with healthier options. But once you get used to choosing legumes, eggs, chicken, protein-rich grains, or other types of plant-based protein, you may find that following the gout diet allows you to feel full and satisfied. (Reduced gout symptoms and attacks can also be strong motivators for change.)

Weight Loss

Again, many studies have shown that reaching and maintaining a healthy weight is one way to reduce the frequency of gout flare-ups. But if you plan to lose weight, avoid crash diets. By losing weight too quickly, you may end up triggering an attack.

As with all dietary plans, a slow and steady approach is better for your health and something you'll be better able to maintain over the long run.

Exercise and General Health

In addition to following the gout diet, your healthcare provider may recommend that you make other changes to help you live comfortably with gout. The recommendations may include physical activity.

Studies have shown that regular exercise can help to improve joint function and help you to maintain a healthy weight. However, strenuous exercise can do more harm than good and dehydration may raise the level of uric acid in serum and trigger gout.

7 Days Gout-Friendly Diet Eating Plan

Eating a gout-friendly diet will help you relieve the pain and swelling, while preventing future attacks.

Here is a sample gout-friendly menu for one week.

Monday

• Breakfast: Oats with Greek yogurt and 1/4 cup (about 31 grams) berries.

• Lunch: Quinoa salad with boiled eggs and fresh veggies.

- Dinner: Whole wheat pasta with roasted chicken, spinach, bell peppers and low-fat feta cheese.

Tuesday

- Breakfast: Smoothie with 1/2 cup (74 grams) blueberries, 1/2 cup (15 grams) spinach, 1/4 cup (59 ml) Greek yogurt and 1/4 cup (59 ml) low-fat milk.

- Lunch: Whole grain sandwich with eggs and salad.

- Dinner: Stir-fried chicken and vegetables with brown rice.

Wednesday

- Breakfast: Overnight oats — 1/3 cup (27 grams) rolled oats, 1/4 cup (59 ml) Greek yogurt, 1/3 cup (79 ml) low-fat milk, 1 tbsp (14 grams) chia seeds, 1/4 cup (about 31 grams) berries and 1/4 tsp (1.2 ml) vanilla extract. Let sit overnight.

• Lunch: Chickpeas and fresh vegetables in a whole wheat wrap.

• Dinner: Herb-baked salmon with asparagus and cherry tomatoes.

Thursday

• Breakfast: Overnight chia seed pudding — 2 tbsp (28 grams) chia seeds, 1 cup (240 ml) Greek yogurt and 1/2 tsp (2.5 ml) vanilla extract with sliced fruits of your choice. Let sit in a bowl or mason jar overnight.

• Lunch: Leftover salmon with salad.

- Dinner: Quinoa, spinach, eggplant and feta salad.

Friday

- Breakfast: French toast with strawberries.

- Lunch: Whole grain sandwich with boiled eggs and salad.

- Dinner: Stir-fried tofu and vegetables with brown rice.

Saturday

- Breakfast: Mushroom and zucchini frittata.

- Lunch: Leftover stir-fried tofu and brown rice.

- Dinner: Homemade chicken burgers with a fresh salad.

Sunday

- Breakfast: Two-egg omelet with spinach and mushrooms.

- Lunch: Chickpeas and fresh vegetables in a whole wheat wrap.

- Dinner: Scrambled egg tacos — scrambled eggs with spinach and bell peppers on whole wheat tortillas.

GOUT DIET RECIPES

In this part are nutritional gout diet recipes tp put your gout at bay.

Gout Safe Vegetable Soup

Preparation time

2 hours 30 minutes

Ingredients

Homemade Vegetarian Broth

- 1 Tablespoon Oil

- 2 each leeks

- 2 each carrots

- 2 ribs celery I used four tops with leaves

- 1/4 teaspoon salt

- 8 Cups water

Soup

- 1 Tablespoon Oil

- 2 Cups Potatoes Diced

- 1 Cups Mushrooms Diced

- 1.5 Cups Cauliflower Diced

- 1 Cup Onion Diced

- 1 Cup Celery Diced

- 1 Cup Carrot Diced

- 1 Tablespoon Garlic Minced

- 1.5 Cups Red Beans cooked

- 2 sprigs Rosemary

- 4 sprigs Thyme

- 2 Cups Spinach.

Instructions

Homemade Vegetarian Broth

1. To a pot on medium heat add one Tablespoon of oil and two leeks that have been cut up.

2. Cook for about three minutes until they start to soften up.

3. To a pot on medium heat add one Tablespoon of oil and two leeks that have been cut up.

4. Cook for about three minutes until they start to soften up.

5. Add two carrots that have been cut up. Mine were peeled so they would look good in the photo but that is optional.

6. Add two carrots that have been cut up. Mine were peeled so they would look good in the photo but that is optional.

7. Add the top of a few celery stalks with leaves.

8. Add the top of a few celery stalks with leaves.

9. Cover with water (I used 8 cups) add 1/4 teaspoon of salt.

10. Bring to a simmer and cook until the carrots are very tender but not quite mush. This took me one hour.

11. Then turn off the heat and let it cool down a little. Cover with water (I used 8 cups) add 1/4 teaspoon of salt.

12. Bring to a simmer and cook until the carrots are very tender but not quite mush. This took me one hour.

13. Then turn off the heat and let it cool down a little.

14. When the broth has cool to a safe to handle tempature strain out the veggies. For this I used a strainer lined with cheesecloth.

15. When the broth has cool to a safe to handle tempature strain out the veggies. For this I used a strainer lined with cheesecloth.

16. Remove the carrots and set aside.

17. Then squeeze most of the liquid out of the leeks and celery. This gave me six and a half cups of liquid.

18. Remove the carrots and set aside.

19. Then squeeze most of the liquid out of the leeks and celery. This gave me six and a half cups of liquid.

Soup

1. Add the carrots to some of the broth and blend. I used a stick blender. You could just dump all of the broth in a blender with the carrots and blend. But this stick blender is new and I wanted to give a test drive. Doing this gives the stock some body and a nice color. You could blend all of the veggies but then you would need to strain it. Add the carrots to some of the broth and blend. I used a stick blender. You could just dump all of the broth in a blender with the carrots and blend. But this stick blender is new and I wanted to give a test drive. Doing this gives the stock some body and a nice color. You could blend all of the veggies but then you would need to strain it.

2. With a pot on medium heat add one tablespoon of oil the onions, raw carrots, celery and garlic.

3. Cook until the onions are translucent (approximately three to five minutes).

4. With a pot on medium heat add one tablespoon of oil the onions, raw carrots, celery and garlic.

5. Cook until the onions are translucent (approximately three to five minutes).

6. When the onions are translucent add the broth, potatoes and the herbs.

7. Bring to a simmer and cook ten minutes.

8. When the onions are translucent add the broth, potatoes and the herbs. Bring to a

9. simmer and cook ten minutes.

10. Add the cauliflower and red beans.

11. Simmer another five minutes.

12. Add the cauliflower and red beans.

13. Simmer another five minutes.

14. Add the package of frozen green beans and cook until the potatoes and cauliflower are tender (approximately another five minutes).

15. Add the package of frozen green beans and cook until the potatoes and cauliflower are tender (approximately another five minutes).

16. At the end of cooking add two cups of spinach.

Potato (or Caulflower) Leek Soup

Preparation time

30 minutes

Ingredients

• 3 tablespoons unsalted grass-fed butter, ghee or coconut oil

• 4 washed leeks, white AND green parts, roughly chopped (crazy me, don't mind the green...Julia is rolling in her grave)

• 3 cloves garlic, peeled and smashed (no need to mince since you'll be blending to finish)

• ¾ cup of cooking sherry

- 2 lbs yukon or russet potatoes, (cauliflower for paleo) scrubbed/washed well and roughly chopped into ½-inch pieces

- 8 cups bone broth or chicken stock or veggie stock

- 2 bay leaves

- 1½ teaspoons finely chopped fresh thyme

- 1 teaspoon sea salt

- ¼ teaspoon ground black pepper

- 1 cup plain cashew cream (to replace heavy dairy cream)

- 2 tablespoons Braggs (with the mother!) apple cider vinegar

- ¾ cup of nutritional yeast (great source of protein)

- Chives, finely chopped (optional)

- Bacon, chopped in small cubes (optional)

- Grated asiago cheese (optional)

- Chili Oil (optional for drizzling)

Instructions

1. Melt the butter over medium heat in a large dutch oven. (Just my preference for making soups.)

2. Add the leeks and garlic and to simmer, stirring regularly, until soft and wilted, about 10 minutes.

3. No browning allowed, but sherry splashing to deglaze encouraged.

4. Add the potatoes (or separately steamed and drained cauliflower), stock/broth of choice, bay leaves, thyme, salt and pepper to pot and bring to a slow boil.

5. Cover and turn the heat down to low.

6. Simmer for 20 minutes, or until the potatoes are very soft and break apart when smooshed with a fork.

7. If using cauliflower ou can immediately blend after adding it COOKED into the broth mixture.

8. Fish out bay leaves, then add the nutritional yeast and purée the soup with a hand-held immersion blender until smooth. (Alternatively, use a standard blender to purée the soup in batches but that's a pain in the ass.)

9. Add the cashew cream and apple cider vinegar and bring to a simmer.

10. Taste and adjust seasoning with salt and pepper.

11. Garnish whichever way you like! This makes a great weeknight meal with grilled sandwiches done on the panini press.

Gout and Joint Pain Juice

Preparation time

5 minutes

Ingredients

- 1 medium-sized cucumber, roughly chopped

- 2 ribs of celery, rinsed

- 1/2 of a lemon

- 1 -inch piece ginger root, peeled

Instructions

1. One by one, place all of the ingredients through the juicer.

2. Once you are finished, drink the juice.

3. It may be beneficial to drink this juice once a day.

Tart Cherry-Apple Crunch

Preparation time

40 minutes

Ingredients

- 1 pound frozen pitted tart cherries

- 1 green apple, cored and diced

- 1/4 cup light brown sugar, packed

- 1/2 teaspoon almond extract

- 1 1/2 tablespoons cornstarch or arrowroot powder

- 1/2 cup unsweetened cherry or apple juice

- Nonstick cooking spray

Topping:

- 1/4 cup old-fashioned rolled oats

- 1/4 cup brown sugar

- 1/4 cup walnuts, chopped

- 2 tablespoons whole-wheat pastry flour

- 3 tablespoons grapeseed oil

- 1/4 teaspoon salt (optional)

Instructions

1. Preheat oven to 400°F.

2. In a bowl, toss together the cherries, apple, brown sugar, and almond extract.

3. In a cup, mix the cornstarch and juice and add to the fruit mixture, stirring well.

4. Pour the mixture into an 8-inch-square baking dish sprayed with nonstick cooking spray.

5. Mix together the remaining ingredients.

6. Crumble the mixture on top of the fruit.

7. Bake for 30 minutes.

8. Raise heat to a broil and brown topping lightly for 1-2 minutes.

9. Remove from oven.

10. Serve warm or cold.

One Pot Chicken And Lentil Stew

Preparation time

1 hour

INGREDIENTS

- 1 cup dried green lentils

- 2 medium raw chicken breasts, cut into 1 inch cubes (thawed chicken breasts work great as well!)

- 1/2 tsp celery seed

- 1/2 tsp coriander

- 1 tsp paprika

- 1 tsp Italian seasoning

- 1 5.3 oz container of plain greek yogurt, reserving a few tbsp to dollop on top at the end.

- 1/2 small orange, juiced (squeezing the juice out is fine)

- 1 tbsp olive oil or coconut oil

- 1 red onion, chopped (or yellow/white onion, whatever you have)

- 3/4 cup coconut milk

- 3/4 cup chicken broth

- 1/4 tsp salt

- pinch of pepper

- parsley or cilantro as garnish

INSTRUCTIONS

1. Boil about 3 cups of water in a pot. Salt the water.

2. Toss in 1 cup of dried green lentils and boil for two minutes.

3. Remove from heat. Keeping the lentils in the water, let them soak for 1 hour.

4. Make your chicken marinade: Place chicken cubes in a bowl and add in celery seed, 1/2 tsp coriander, paprika and Italian seasoning.

5. Empty almost the entire greek yogurt cup, reserving a few tbsp to dollop on top at the end.

6. Squeeze in the juice of 1/2 of an orange and stir to combine all ingredients.

7. Place a lid or plastic wrap over the top and refrigerate for at least 10 minutes, up to 2 hours.

8. While the chicken is marinating, and once the lentils have sat in their water for 1 hour, drain the lentils and pick through, discarding any extra hard lentils or debris.

9. Heat a medium to large cast iron dutch oven over medium high heat and add 1 tbsp of olive oil or coconut oil.

10. Add in your marinated chicken and cook undisturbed for about 5 minutes.

11. Toss in your chopped red onion, flip the chicken and continue to cook for another 5 minutes, undisturbed.

12. Add in your previously soaked green lentils, coconut milk, chicken broth and salt/pepper.

13. Stir to fully combine, place the lid on the pot and simmer for 35 minutes, stirring occasionally.

14. Once done, scoop lentils and chicken out into a bowl using a slotted spoon.

15. Garnish with parsley and a dollop of plain Greek yogurt and enjoy! You can use the left over liquid as the base for a sauce, or you can freeze it and use it later!

Lemon Chicken with Carrots, Parsnips and Leeks

Preparation time

1 hour

Ingredients

- 2 chicken breasts

- 1 onion

- 1 bunch soup vegetables (plus other aromatic vegetables such as celery or onion)

- ½ small lemon

- 1 tablespoonvegetable oil

- salt

- 2 black peppercorns

- 1 bay leaf

- 2 lime leaves

- 2 cloves

- 2 allspice

- 1 kohlrabi

- 3 waxy potatoes

- 4 ounces peas (frozen)

Instructions

1. Rinse chicken breasts and pat dry with paper towels.

2. Lemon Chicken with Carrots, Parsnips and Leeks preparation step 2

3. Halve an unpeeled onion.

4. Lemon Chicken with Carrots, Parsnips and Leeks preparation step 3

5. From soup vegetables, peel carrots and parsley root.

6. Trim leeks and celery.

7. Chop 1 carrot, half of the parsley root, half of the celery and the greens of the leeks.

8. Pluck some of the celery leaves, rinse and set aside.

9. Lemon Chicken with Carrots, Parsnips and Leeks preparation step 4

10. Rinse the lemon in hot water, then cut into slices.

11. In a pot coated with oil, sear the onion halves over high heat, remove from pan.

12. In the same pot coated with oil, cook the chicken breasts over medium heat.

13. Turn as needed for even cooking.

14. Lemon Chicken with Carrots, Parsnips and Leeks preparation step 6

15. Add the onion halves, chopped soup vegetables and celery leaves to the pot.

16. Pour in approximately 2 cups of water and bring to a quick boil.

17. Add salt, peppercorns, bay leaf, lime leaves, cloves, allspice berries, and lemon slices.

18. Simmer for about 20 minutes with the lid ajar.

19. Lemon Chicken with Carrots, Parsnips and Leeks preparation step 7

20. Meanwhile, roughly chop the rest of the soup vegetables.

21. Scrub and peel potatoes and kohlrabi and cut into uniform pieces.

22. Remove chicken from the pot and set aside.

23. Lemon Chicken with Carrots, Parsnips and Leeks preparation step 9

24. Pour cooking liquid through a fine sieve into another pot.

25. Season with salt and pepper to taste.

26. Lemon Chicken with Carrots, Parsnips and Leeks preparation step 10

27. Over medium heat, bring potatoes and remaining soup vegetables to a simmer.

28. Cook for about 15 minutes.

29. Lemon Chicken with Carrots, Parsnips and Leeks preparation step 11

30. Add peas and chicken and simmer for another 5 minutes.

31. Using a slotted spoon, transfer vegetables from the pot onto plates.

32. Top each plate with a little broth.

33. Arrange chicken over the vegetable broth. Sprinkle with reserved chopped celery leaves and serve.

Paleo Grilled Chicken

Preparation time

3 hours

INGREDIENTS

- 2 pounds chicken breasts boneless and skinless

- 8 cups water

- 3 tbsp salt

- 2 cloves garlic whole

- 2 tbsp coconut aminos or soy sauce

- 1 bay leaf

- 1 tsp coriander seeds ((whole))

- 1 tsp cumin seeds ((whole))

- 1 tsp black peppercorns ((whole))

- 1 tbsp cumin ((ground))

- 1 tbsp curry powder

- 1 tbsp chili powder

- 1/2 tbsp ground allspice ((ground))

- 1/2 tsp ground cinnamon ((ground))

- 1 tsp black pepper ((ground))

INSTRUCTIONS

Brining Instructions:

1. Brine. Pour water into a large ziplock bag. Add in salt, garlic, coconut aminos, bay leaf, coriander seeds, cumin seeds and peppercorns. Give mixture enough time for the salt to dissolve.

2. Chill. Place chicken breasts into bag and put in fridge for 2 hours.

3. Rinse. Remove the bag from the fridge; rinse the chicken.

4. Drain. Place chicken into sieve and let it drain.

5. Spice Blend & Grilling Directions:

6. Mix. Mix the spices, stirring together with a fork in a small bowl.

7. Preheat grill on high heat for about 10 minutes (with lid closed)

8. Rub. Rub the chicken pieces in the seasoning mix, massaging it as you go.

9. The more coating that sticks, the more flavor!

10. Grill. Put the chicken on the preheated grill (smooth side down). With the lid closed, cook for about 4 minutes.

11. Flip chicken, cook for another 4 minutes (or until chicken is browned) and make sure chicken is cooked through.

12. Serve. Remove from grill and enjoy!

Slow Cooker Vegetarian Chili

Preparation time

30 minutes

Ingredients

- 2 tablespoons vegetable oil

- 1 yellow onion

- 3 cloves garlic

- 1 green bell pepper

- 2 carrots

- 2 small zucchini

- 1 cup diced walnuts

- 28 oz can pinto beans

- 28 oz can diced tomatoes

- 2 tablespoons chili powder

- 1 tablespoon dried oregano

- 1 tablespoon dried basil

- 1 teaspoon cinnamon

- 1 teaspoon cumin

- 1+ teaspoon salt

- 1 teaspoon cocoa powder

- Avocado for garnish

Instructions

1. Step one of any delicious chili is to spice the vegetables first.

2. Just like with a curry, it's essential that you sauté the veggies and thoroughly spice them first in order to develop maximum flavor.

3. So first, prep all the vegetables – dice the onion (but save a small piece for garnish), mince the garlic, chop the bell pepper, slice the carrots, slice the zucchini, and chop the walnuts into fairly small pieces.

4. Then, heat a large skillet with a drizzle of vegetable oil and add everything from step one into the pan and allow it to cook 4-5 minutes until the onions become translucent.

5. Add half of the chili powder (1 tablespoon), a teaspoon each of cinnamon and cumin, and a few pinches of salt.

6. Cook for another 4-5 minutes until you have something that looks and smells delicious (and would make great veggie taco filling on its own):

Vegetarian_Chili_Preparation

1. Finally, add this into your slow cooker along with all the other ingredients – diced tomatoes, pinto beans, the remainder of the chili powder, dried basil and oregano, cocoa powder, and a bit more salt.

Note: Don't drain the tomatoes or pinto beans – they will add just the right amount of liquid to this chili.

2. Set your slow cooker to low/medium, walk away, and let this cook for at least 6 hours.

3. Before serving, give the soup a taste and feel free to adjust the seasoning: you can add a little more salt or spices to boost the flavor if needed.

4. Serving with a slice or two of avocado and just a taste of finely-diced raw onions is absolutely not optional.

Veggie Enchiladas

Preparation time

30 minutes

Ingredients:

- 2 corn tortillas

- 1 cup frozen kale

- 1/2 cup frozen corn

- 1 cup enchilada sauce (link to recipe at the bottom)

- 1/2 cup beans (I like black beans, use your favorite)

- 4 tablespoons cashew cream (link to recipe at the bottom)

- 2 tablespoons nutritional yeast

- 1 teaspoon lime juice

- 1/4 teaspoon garlic granules

- salt and pepper (to taste)

- fresh cilantro (garnish)

Instructions:

1. Take the tortillas out of the fridge and let them come to room temperature while you are doing the other prep.

2. Thaw the kale and corn in a large bowl filled with cold water, then drain them and squeeze

out the excess water. This should only take a few minutes.

3. Put the kale and corn back into the bowl.

4. Add the beans to the bowl and mix in 2 tablespoons of cashew cream, all of the nutritional yeast, lime juice and garlic powder.

5. Taste the mixture and add a little salt and pepper if desired.

6. Pour the enchilada sauce into a wide, shallow bowl and dip the tortillas into the liquid so they are coated on all sides with sauce.

7. Fill each tortilla with half of the kale mixture, then roll and set into a baking dish with the seam-side down.

8. Make sure to use a baking dish the correct size for the number of enchiladas you are making. A 5x7 dish is perfect for 2, while a 7x10 dish is best for 4-6.

9. Once the torillas are filled and tucked into the dish, pour enchilada sauce on top of them until they are covered. If there isn't enough sauce just add a little water.

10. Bake at 350ºF/180ºC for 20 minutes.

11. Remove from the oven and let cool for 5 minutes before serving.

12. Then drizzle the remaining 2 tablespoons cashew cream across the top and garnish with fresh cilantro.

SUPERFOODS SALAD

Preparation time

15 minutes

INGREDIENTS

- 1 1/2 cup Shredded Carrots

- 1 1/2 cup Broccoli Slaw

- 1 1/2 cup Mukimame or deshelled Edamame

- 1 1/2 cup Blueberry

- 64 Cashews 16 per serving

- 1 cup Walnuts 12 to 14 halves per serving

- 1/4 cup hulled Sunflower Seeds

- 1/2 cup Dried Cranberry

LEMON-GINGER VINAIGRETTE

- 1 large Ripe Lemon squeeze as much as you can (if the lemon is smaller, you can use 2)

- 1/4 cup Olive Oil

- 3 tbsp. Apple Cider Vinegar or red wine vinegar

- 1 inch Fresh Ginger grated

- 1 teaspoon minced Garlic

- 1 teaspoon Dried Parsley

- 1/4 teaspoon Chili Powder

- Himalayan Salt to taste

INSTRUCTIONS

1. Wash all the vegetables and fruit, then prepare them by slicing, shredding, and grating.

2. Slice Kale into bite size pieces, and place in the large bowl.

3. Mix everything for lemon-ginger vinaigrette in the glass jar with a fitted lid and season with salt to taste, start with 1/4 teaspoon and taste.

4. Close the lid and shake the jar to combine all the ingredients.

5. Pour the vinaigrette over the kale and massage it for about one minute or until the kale is tender.

6. Squeeze the kale using your hands. You will end up with half of the size in the bowl. You got to do this step to make kale tastier.

7. Now add all the other ingredients (fruits and vegetables) and lightly toss with the kale.

8. Taste and see if you need to add a pinch or two of Salt.

9. Serve just a salad immediately or place in the container/jar with a fitted lid and keep in the fridge for up to 2 days.

CHICKEN BROCCOLI CASSEROLE WITH CHERRIES AND ALMONDS

Preparation time

35 minutes

Ingredients

- 1 large head of broccoli cut into bite-size florets (or buy a large bag of broccoli florets)

- 3 tablespoons olive oil

- 1 teaspoon salt

- 1 teaspoon pepper

- 3 cloves garlic, minced

- 1/3 cup chicken stock (use more if your think your mixture seems dry)

- 2 chicken breasts cooked and shredded (I used a rotisserie chicken!)

- 1 cup plain Greek yogurt

- 6 ounces Feta cheese

- 4 green onions, chopped

- 1/3 cup sliced almonds, toasted

- ½ cup dried tart cherries

INSTRUCTIONS

1. Preheat oven to 425F.

2. Clean and cut broccoli florets into bite-sized pieces, drizzle with olive oil, and sprinkle with salt and pepper.

3. Bake in a 9 X 13 baking dish for 10 minutes at 425 degrees.

4. While the broccoli is roasting, shred the chicken and set it aside.

5. Heat up a medium-sized skillet on the stove, add olive oil and minced garlic. Cook for 1 minute then add the chicken stock, and bring to a simmer.

6. Add the chicken and stir.

7. Fold in the Greek yogurt, 3 ounces of the feta cheese, green onions, half the cherries and half the almonds.

8. When the broccoli is finished roasting, turn the oven temp down to 375, and fold the chicken mixture into the baking dish with the broccoli.

9. Then sprinkle with the

10. remaining feta, almonds and cherries.

11. Bake for 15-20 minutes covered, and serve.

Curried Carrot, Sweet Potato, and Ginger Soup

Preparation time

35 minutes

Ingredients

- 2 teaspoons canola oil

- 1/2 cup chopped shallots

- 3 cups (1/2-inch) cubed peeled sweet potato

- 1 1/2 cups (1/4-inch) sliced peeled carrots

- 1 tablespoon grated ginger

- 2 teaspoons curry powder

- 3 cups fat-free, less-sodium chicken broth

- 1/2 teaspoon salt

Instructions

1. Heat oil in a large saucepan over medium-high heat.

2. Add shallots; saute 3 minutes or until tender.

3. Add potato, carrots, ginger, and curry; cook 2 minutes.

4. Add broth; bring to a boil.

5.   Cover, reduce heat, and simmer 25 minutes or until vegetables are tender; stir in salt.

6. Pour half of soup in a food processor; pulse until smooth.

7.   Repeat procedure with remaining soup.

Waldorf Salad

Preparation time

10 minutes

Ingredients

- 2 tablespoons low-fat mayonnaise

- 1 tablespoon lemon juice

- 2 small (Gala or Fuji) apples, cubed

- 1 cup seedless red grapes, halved

- 1/3 cup dried cranberries

- 1/4 cup coarsely chopped walnuts

- 1/4 cup thinly sliced celery (about 1 stalk)

- 8 Boston or Bibb lettuce leaves

Instructions

1. Combine mayonnaise and lemon juice in a medium bowl.

2. Add apples, grapes, and cranberries; mix well.

3. Add the walnuts and celery, and mix well.

4. Serve it on a bed of 2 lettuce leaves.

5. The salad can be refrigerated up to 2 hours before serving.

Warm Eggplant and Goat Cheese Sandwiches

Preparation time

22 minutes

Ingredients

- 1 teaspoon olive oil

- 2 (1/4-inch) vertical slices small eggplant

- Cooking spray

- 1/4 teaspoon salt

- 1/4 teaspoon freshly ground black pepper

- 1/4 cup (2 ounces) goat cheese, softened

- 2 (1 1/2-ounce) rustic sandwich rolls

- 2 (1/4-inch) slices tomato

- 1 cup Arugula

Instructions

1. Preheat oven to 275°.

2. Brush oil over eggplant

3. Heat a large nonstick skillet coated with cooking spray over medium-high heat.

4. Add eggplant; cook 5 minutes on each side or until lightly browned.

5. Sprinkle with salt and pepper.

6. Spread about 1 tablespoon of goat cheese over cut side of each roll half.

7. Place rolls on a baking sheet, cheese sides up; bake at 275° for 8 to 10 minutes or until thoroughly heated.

8. Remove from oven; top bottom half of each roll with 1 eggplant slice, 1 tomato slice, and 1/2 cup arugula.

9. Top sandwiches with top halves of rolls.

Frying Pan Frittata

Preparation time

20 minutes

Ingredients

- ½ small onion, chopped

- 1 cup red and green peppers, sliced thin or chopped small

- 4 cups spinach and/or other leafy greens, torn or chopped (1 cup if using frozen)

- 1 tbsp extra-virgin olive oil or canola oil

- 1/4 tsp garlic powder

- 1/4 tsp black pepper

- 1/2 tsp dried oregano and/or basil (or 2 tablespoons of chopped fresh herbs)

- 4 eggs

Instructions

1. Use a medium-sized frying pan over medium heat and heat oil until shiny.

2. Add the onion, stirring until just soft

3. Add the peppers.

4. Stir until the onions and peppers are very soft and just browning.

5. Add the spinach/greens to the pan and stir until wilted and hot.

6. Crack the eggs into a bowl and whisk them up with a fork until they're uniformly yellow and a little foamy.

7. Pour the eggs over all the veggies, turn the heat to low, and cover the pan.

8. Shake the pan a few times during cooking, which more evenly distributes the eggs and prevents sticking.

9. Check frittata after three to four minutes.

10. If the eggs look done, loosen it with a spatula to make sure there is no runniness. If there is, cook thirty seconds to a minute longer, covered.

11. Using a spatula, slide frittata gently onto a large plate and serve. We slice this up like a pizza.

Plant-Based Mushroom Soup

Preparation time

1 hour 5 minutes

Ingredients

- 2 red onions finely chopped

- 4 garlic cloves crushed then finely chopped

- 1 large potato peeled and chopped into small, equal pieces

- 15 g fresh thyme leaves only, discard the stalks

- 50 g dried porcini mushrooms (follow packet instructions, but they're usually soaked in

500ml/1 pint boiling water for 30 minutes. Remove the porcini from the liquid for the soup and keep the water/stock/liquid for the soup as well)

• 259 g closed cap chestnut mushrooms roughly chopped

• 150 g closed cap white mushrooms

• 1 litre pints stock

• 28 g fresh flat leaved parsley keep a few leaves whole and finely chop the remainder

• 1 zest of one lemon and half of its juice

Instructions

1. Add two inches of water to a large pot.

2. Add the onions, garlic, potato and thyme to the pot.

3. Bring to a fast bubble, then turn down and simmer for approximately 10 minutes with the lid on.

4. Make sure that the mixture does not catch on. If it does, add some more cold water.

5. Add the porcini with their soaking water to the pot with all the other mushrooms. Stir well. Cook for 20 minutes with the lid off.

6. Add the stock and cook for a further 20 minutes.

7. Add the finely chopped parsley then whizz with a hand blender or a countertop blender until smooth.

8. Mix the lemon juice zest with half of the lemon juice.

9. Serve the mushroom soup into warm soup bowls with a swirl of the lemon juice and zest and a scattering of some of the reserved parsley.

Asparagus salad with roasted sweet potato, avocado and energetic green pesto.

Preparation time

40 minutes

Ingredients

Salad

- 1/2 bunch asparagus (you can splash with colors - today i used white)

- 1 medium sweet potato

- 4-5 cocktail tomatoes

- 1/2 piece avocado

To bake a potato (to be emptied) we need: dried or fresh rosemary, Himalayan salt, freshly ground pepper and olive oil

Energetic green pesto.

- 1/2 bunch parsley

- 2 Tbsp hemp oil (if you can not use cold pressed flaxseed oil)

- 2 tbsp lemon juice or apple cider vinegar

- 1 tbsp molasses (or alternatively agave syrup)

- Himalayan salt, freshly ground pepper to taste

Instructions

Salad

1. Sweet potato is thoroughly washed with a brush - we do not peel from the skin, not to deprive it of the most important nutrients and cut into slices. We put on a plate, salt, pepper, rosemary and gently sprinkle with olive oil. We bake in the oven with the upper baking approx. 10-15 min. At 180 degrees.

2. Asparagus gently wash and if they have a thicker skin gently peel from half down.

3. Boil steam until tender, but not overcooked (about 10-15 minutes depending on the thickness of the asparagus).

4. On the plate we put asparagus, baked sliced sweet potatoes, cut in half a cocktail, add cherry tomatoes and pesto water all.

5. Before serving, let the salad gently sprinkle with a little salt, pepper and chopped chives, which will give the dish a distinct flavor.

Energetic green pesto

1. Parsley leaves are washed thoroughly, dried and finely chopped (this will help us prepare the pesto).

2. Blend all ingredients and mix to get a paste.

Chicken Veggie Stir Fry

Preparation time

Ingredients

- 2 tablespoons reduced-sodium soy sauce, divided

- 1 tablespoon minced fresh ginger

- Juice of 1 lime, divided

- 2 teaspoons sesame oil, divided

- 1 pound skinless, boneless chicken breast, cut into bite-size pieces

- 1 tablespoon expeller pressed canola oil

- 2 carrots, cut into very thin rounds (about 1 cup)

- 2 cups bite-size broccoli florets (from 1 small bunch)

- 1 medium zucchini, cut in half lengthwise and then cut into ¼-inch-thick half moons (about 2 cups)

- 4 garlic cloves, minced

- 2 green onions cut into ¼-inch pieces (white and green parts)

- 1 jalapeño pepper, seeded and minced

- ¼ cup sliced fresh basil

- ¼ cup chopped fresh cilantro

- Brown rice, optional

Instructions

1. Place 1 tablespoon of the soy sauce, ginger, juice of half a lime, and 1 teaspoon of the sesame oil in a large zip-top plastic bag or bowl.

2. Add the chicken pieces, seal the bag, and refrigerate for 1 hour or up to 24 hours.

3. When ready to make your stir fry, heat the oil in a large wok or nonstick skillet over medium-high heat.

4. Add the chicken and the marinade and stir fry for 1 minute.

5. Add the carrots, broccoli, zucchini, garlic, green onions, and jalapeno pepper and stir fry 7

more minutes, or until the chicken is done and the vegetables are crisp tender.

6. Stir in the remaining 1 tablespoon soy sauce, remaining lime juice, and the remaining sesame oil.

7. Before serving, stir in the basil and cilantro.

8. Serve with brown rice as desired.

Slow Cooker Chicken With Honey, Garlic and Sesame

Preparation time

4 hours 20 minutes

INGREDIENTS

- 12 pieces chicken thighs, drumsticks, legs

- 2 tbsp honey best to chose local honey

- 4 tbsp chicken broth or water

- 1/4 cup tamari coconut aminos can be used as a replacement

- 3 cloves garlic pressed

- 1 tsp smoked chili pepper smoked paprika can be used as a replacement

- 2 tsp dried oregano

- 2 tbsp unfiltered apple cider vinegar

- 2 tsp Worcestershire sauce

- 1 tbsp toasted sesame oil

INSTRUCTIONS

1. Mix all ingredients in a bowl, then place into the base of the slow cooker.

2. Place chicken on top and mix in sauce.

3. Cook on low for 4 hrs.

4. Serve over your favorite veggies and rice or quinoa if using.

Baked Ziti with Roasted Vegetables

Preparation time

1 hour 20 minutes

INGREDIENTS

Roasted veggies

• 1 medium head of cauliflower, cut into bite-sized florets

• 1 red bell pepper, cut into 1" squares

• 1 medium yellow onion, sliced into wedges about ½" wide

- 2 tablespoons extra-virgin olive oil, divided

- ¼ teaspoon fine sea salt, divided

Pasta and everything else

- 8 ounces ziti, rigatoni or penne pasta

- 4 cups (32 ounces) marinara sauce (homemade or store-bought), divided

- ¼ cup chopped fresh basil, plus extra for garnish

- 8 ounces (2 packed cups) grated part-skim mozzarella cheese, divided

- 2 cups (16 ounces) cottage cheese or ricotta cheese, divided

INSTRUCTIONS

1. To roast the veggies: Preheat the oven to 425 degrees Fahrenheit with racks in the middle and upper third of the oven.

2. Line two large, rimmed baking sheets with parchment paper to prevent the vegetables from sticking.

3. Place the cauliflower florets on one pan.

4. On the other pan, combine the bell peppers and onion.

5. Drizzle half of the olive oil over one pan, and the other half over the other pan. Sprinkle the salt over the two pans.

6. Gently toss until the vegetables on each pan are lightly coated in oil.

7. Arrange the vegetables in an even layer across each pan.

8. Bake until the vegetables are tender and caramelized on the edges, about 30 to 35 minutes, tossing the veggies and swapping their rack positions halfway (lower rack to upper rack, and vice versa).

9. Leave the oven on at 425, because we're going to bake the dish at the same temperature.

10. If you end up with any stray burnt onion pieces, discard them, and set the vegetables aside.

11. Meanwhile, bring a large pot of salted water to boil.

12. Cook the pasta just until al dente, according to package directions (it will continue to cook

while it bakes in the oven, so you want the pasta to still have a little bite to it).

13. Drain and return the pasta to the pot.

14. Add 2 cups of the marinara, the chopped basil, and ½ cup of the mozzarella to the pasta. Gently stir to combine.

15. It's assembly time! Spread 1 cup of additional marinara sauce inside a 9×13" baker.

16. Top with half of the pasta mixture, and gently spread it into an even layer.

17. Evenly sprinkle the roasted cauliflower on top, then dollop 1 cup of the cottage cheese over the cauliflower (it doesn't need to be spread into an even layer), followed by ½ cup of the mozzarella.

18. Top the mozzarella with the remaining pasta.

19. Then sprinkle the roasted peppers and onion on top, dollop the remaining cup of ricotta on top, then dollop the remaining cup of marinara on that, then sprinkle the remaining cheese all over.

20. Place a clean, rimmed baking sheet on the lower oven rack to catch any drippings.

21. Place the ziti, uncovered, on top of the baking sheet.

22. Bake for 30 minutes, then transfer to the upper rack for 2 to 5 more minutes until the cheese is deeply golden, if desired.

23. Remove the baker from the oven and let it cool for 10 minutes before serving (trust me).

Sprinkle freshly torn basil on top, slice with a sharp knife, and serve.

Egg and Sausage Breakfast Sandwich

Preparation time

15 minutes

Ingredients

nonstick cooking spray

- 1/4 cup liquid low-cholesterol egg substitute

- 1 English muffin

- 1 turkey sausage patty

- 1 tablespoon shredded natural sharp cheddar cheese

Instructions

1. In a small skillet sprayed with nonstick cooking spray, pour egg product and cook over medium low heat.

2. When egg appears almost cooked through, turn over with a spatula and cook additional 30 seconds.

3. Toast English muffin.

4. Place turkey sausage patty on a plate, cover with a paper towel and cook in the microwave for 1 minute or the time recommended on package.

5. Assemble cooked egg on English muffin (fold to fit muffin).

6. Top with sausage patty, then sharp cheddar cheese and remaining muffin half.

Black Beans and Brown Rice

Preparation time

1 hour 35 minutes

Ingredients

Black beans

- 4 cups beans (black) uncooked

- 6 red onions diced

- 1 cup fresh garlic chopped

- 2 tablespoons cumin

- 1 tablespoon coriander

- 1 chipotle pepper remove before serving

- 1-1/2 carrots diced

- 2 teaspoons black pepper freshly ground

- 3 quarts water

- 1/2 bunch cilantro leaves picked and chopped

Brown Rice

- 2 cups rice (brown) uncooked

- 1/2 cup onions diced

- 1/2 cup garlic fresh, chopped

- 1/2 teaspoon black pepper freshly ground

- 1 tablespoon soy sauce, low sodium

- 2 teaspoons cumin

- 5 cups water

Instructions

Black Beans

1. Soak beans overnight, rinse, and drain.

2. In a large stockpot, bring to a boil all ingredients for black bean part of recipe, except cilantro.

3. Then reduce heat, cover, and simmer until beans are soft, about 1-1/2 hours.

4. When ready to serve, stir in cilantro.

5. Remove chipotle.

Brown Rice

1. In a large nonstick medium-hot saute pan, saute rice with all ingredients, except water, until garlic starts to brown.

2. Add water & bring to a boil.

3. Reduce heat, cover, and simmer until rice is cooked through, about 40 minutes.

4. When done, combine with cooked black beans, or serve separately.

Chicken Geprek Oatmeal

Preparation time

20 minutes

Ingredients

• 1 chicken breast.

• 1 egg.

• Smooth oatmeal.

• Provide a little oil for frying (canola tropicanaslim).

You need Royco.

• Geprek chili ingredients.

- Prepare 8 bird's eye chilies.

- Prepare 5 curly red chilies.

- You need 2 garlic.

- Prepare 3 shallots.

- Prepare a little salt.

Instructions

1. Wash the chicken thoroughly, then I boil it first so that it cooks evenly after cooking, drain it then add a little royco.

2. Prepare 4 tablespoons of oatmeal and blend until smooth.

3. Wrap the chicken in the egg oatmeal twice, heat the oil just a little, I use canola oil from

tropicanaslim, then fry it until it's cooked or if there is a frying pan you can use it.

4. Don't go back and forth for fear of being crushed.

5. Just turn it once when it turns brown, remove and drain.

6. Prepare clean water and boil the broccoli, drain.

7. Prepare all my chili sauce, fry it in canola oil for a while then grind until smooth.

8. Geprek chicken sprinkled with chili sauce

9. I serve it with red rice mantuls pisan

Fresh Tomatoes and Goat Meat

Preparation time

15 minutes

Ingredients

Prepare Tomatoes

• Make ready Garlic nd ginger

• Get Pepper

• Take Maggi

• Get Salt

• Take leaf Curry

• Prepare Curry and thyme

- Take Onions

- Make ready Goat meat

Instructions

1. Wash ur goat meat nd spice very well for 10mins

2. Put ur tomatoes Inside ur stock and groundnut oil for 5mins

3. Add ur onions curry nd curry leaf ur stew is ready.

4. Come out so lovely

Superfood Anti-Inflammatory Smoothie

Preparation time

5 minutes

Ingredients

- 1/2 can Coconut Milk

- 1 cup Frozen Strawberries

- 1 Tsp Maple Syrup

- 1 Tsp Fresh Ginger

- 1-2oz Tart Cherry Juice

Instructions

1. Through all ingredients in the blender and blend until smooth

Beet, Carrot, and Apple Juice Recipe

Preparation time

20 minutes

Ingredients

- 1 beet root (green tops removed)

- 2 large carrots

- 1 green apple

- 1 inch piece of ginger (peeled, optional)

- 1 tablespoon lemon juice (optional)

Instructions

1. Wash the beet root, carrots, and apple thoroughly, especially if they aren't organic. Use a natural produce wash if possible.

2. Scrub the beets and carrots well.

3. Remove the core and seeds of the apple.

4. If necessary, cut the ingredients into smaller pieces so that they fit into the juicer.

5. Be careful when handling beets — the juice stains everything, so wear gloves if necessary and protect your countertops.

6. Turn on the juicer. Process the first three ingredients, one by one. Juice the ginger root, if you are using it.

7. Stir in the lemon juice, if you are using it.

8. Pour the juice into a glass.

9. Drink immediately or store covered in the refrigerator for up to 24 hours.

10. Stir before drinking. Enjoy!

Baked Sweet Potatoes

Preparation time

50 minutes

Ingredients

- 2 sweet potatoes

- 2 tablespoons of olive oil

- 1 good pinch of salt

- 2 teaspoons of Provence herbs

- 1/2 teaspoon of Espelette pepper

- 1/2 lemon

Instructions

1. In a small ramekin put the olive oil, Provence herbs, Espelette pepper and salt. Mix.

2. Wash the sweet potatoes well.

3. Cut them in half and square the flesh.

4. Lemon them because sweet potatoes oxidize super quickly.

5. Using a brush, brush the sweet potatoes with flavored olive oil.

6. Place them on a baking sheet or a gratin dish and bake in an oven preheated to 180 ° C for 40 minutes of rotating heat.